THE FASCINATING FUNGI

Dr. Farokh J. Master

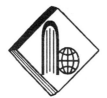

B. Jain Publishers (P) Ltd.

An ISO 9001 : 2000 Certified Company

USA — EUROPE — INDIA

Printed in India

First Edition 1996
Reprint Edition : 1999, 2002 2007

© *Copyright with Publishers*

Publishers by :
B. Jain Publishers Pvt. Ltd.
1921, Street No. 10, Chuna Mandi,
Pahar Ganj, New Delhi - 110 055. (India)
Ph: 2358 0800, 2358 1100, 2358 1300, 2358 3100
Fax: 011-2358 0471; *Email:* bjain@vsnl.com
Website: **www.bjainbooks.com**

Printed in India by
J.J. Offset Printers
522, FIE, Patpar Ganj, Delhi - 110 092
Phones: 2216 9633, 2215 6128

ISBN 978-81-319-0025-3
BOOK CODE : 5184

Dedicated

This book is dedicated to

Dr. B. E. Patel B.Sc. (Hon.), D.M.S. (Cal.)

who stands today as a symbol of dedication

in the hearts of students.

Preface

This book is for those enthusiastic students and practitioners of Homoeopathy who would like to undertake a journey through the world of fungi.

I have tried to explain for the very first time the group symptoms of fungi along with the evolution of mind. In my day to day practice, before I started working on the fungus remedies, my knowledge was limited to using Secale Cor for menorrhagia and Bovista for urticaria, but after a substantial period of indepth study I have perceived the symptomatology of fungal remedies with its differential diagnosis.

The information that is contained in these pages was gathered at my clinic during my practice hours. Dr. Ameet Panchal and Dr. Priya Panchal have contributed a lot observations and suggestions, to whom I am extremely grateful. I am also grateful to Dr. Piroja Bharucha, Dr. Kamal Kodia, Dr. Habibeh Javanmardi and Dr. Niloufer Bamji whose long hours of work are represented in these pages. Without the help of above mentioned people this book would still be just another idea in the mind of a dreamer.

23 - 11 - 1995

Dr. Farokh J. Master
M.D. (Hom.)

VATCHA GANDHY MEMORIAL BLDG.
HUGHES ROAD.
BOMBAY - 400 007.

Contents

1 POISONOUS FUNGI AND FUNGAL POISONS

Since fungi were first used by humans, the poisonous nature of some of them have been recognised. From early on means have been explored to find out whether a fungus contains poison or not, in order to avoid the danger some pose. The reason why some fungi are so dangerous is that unlike any other living thing, fungi are able to assimilate extremely complicated organic compounds. One group of fungi assimilates poisonous substances which attack human organs such as the liver, the kidneys and the blood circulation with potentially fatal consequences. The most dangerous of these fungal poisons are :

1. ∝-amanitin : This is the poison of the bulbous agarics. It leads to the destruction of the liver even in small quantities and is the most frequent cause of fungal poisoning.

2. Orellanin : It leads to protracted poisonings, often with permanent kidney damage.

3. Gyromitrin : This also acts similarly to ∝-amanitin. It is the poison of gyromitra - esculenta turban fungus.

4. Muscarin : This poisonous substance is contained in many species of fungi. It acts as a nerve poison and affects the heart and blood circulation. It can be neutralised by atropine from atropa belladonna. Although it is contained in small doses in amanita pantherina and amanita muscaria the real danger posed by both these fungi is due to other poisonous substances. In addition to those poisons there are many fungi which although they contain no dangerous poisonous substances can cause gastric problems involving several days of sickness.

HEAVY METAL CONTENT

It has been only recently discovered that some naturally growing fungi contain considerable amounts of poisonous heavy metals like lead, quick silver and most of all cadmium. It is not necessary to avoid eating all metal containing fungi especially in view of the fact that other foods particularly liver and kidney contain much higher amounts of these than any fungus. However, a constant consumption of fungi should be avoided particularly of the cadmium rich agaricus.

● ● ●

2 | SHORT SYNOPSIS OF FUNGI

Fungi were regarded as "vapours" of moist soil because they appeared suddenly without allowing observers to see where they originated from; moreover they produced no seeds or fruits and so do not fit into the frame work created for the plant world by the early scientist. Therefore it is not a surprise that fungi were regarded as devilry, the work of dark powers.

We recognise today that an exact fungi identification is guaranteed only by using a microscope. In some particularly difficult groups the identification has to be confirmed by tests for chemical reaction, and even by the investigation of pigments.

What is a Fungus ?

In contrast to more highly evolved plants; fungi do not have chlorophyll and cannot therefore assimilate organic compound. They break up remains of dead plant material and from these compose new organic substances which in turn serve as nutrients for other organisms; In this way fungi fulfil the role of "Waste disposers" in nature. Their work is not only environmentally friendly and clean (of leaves no residue) But they are natural recyclers ensuring that everything has ran its course in nature, can be used once more.

But the role of fungi in nature does not end with this ingenious use of refuse; many fungi combine with the roots of living plants and hence enjoy a symbiotic relationship by obtaining nutrients from the tree root and in turn supply water and salt to its host.

When and where do fungi grow ?

Fungi appear predominantly in late summer and autumn and require a good level of moisture to be able

3

to grow; Species; have specific needs but usually require a preparation time; of two to ten days to form a fruit body. As soon as the first fruit body appears further development proceeds further quickly often in space of a few hours which is true of smaller species; THE AMANITAS are an exception after splitting or tearing the Volva; they only need to extend their stems and expand the cap.

If you notice how many fungus species can appear in the course of few years in a small area; you will realise that some fungi recur seasonally; yet other species can seem to be absent for years and suddenly appear again; not only is the presence of different tree species important but the type of soil as well; some fungus species grow predominantly in old woods others in forest nurseries.

How do fungi Multiply ?

The fungal spores transported locally by air currents or carried by the wind often over large distances form a white wheff (cover of fungal threads) on suitable soils which is called the uni-nucleat mucelium. A precondition for the formation of new fruit bodies is the fusion of mycelia from two wheffs of different lineage. In this process the cells unite but the nucleii remains separate, each cell of a weft capable of fruiting and each cell of a fruit body thus has a two nuclei and a heterothallic mycelium has been found.

The spore production of fungi reaches unimaginary scales e.g.

(1) Gill fungi shed between 25-40 million.

(2) One mature pennybun produces over 10 million spores in a fortnight.

It must be remembered mycelium can survive in the soil and form fruit bodies for centuries.

● ● ●

4

3 | GROUP SYMPTOMS OF FUNGI

NAME OF REMEDIES

1. Agaricus Campestris
2. Agaricus Citrinus
3. Agaricus Emeticus
4. Agaricus Muscaricus
5. Agaricus Pantherinus
6. Agaricus Phalloides
7. Agaricus Procerus
8. Agaricus Semiglobatus
9. Agaricus Strecoranius
10. Boletus Laricis
11. Boletus Luridus
12. Boletus Satanas

13. Bovista Nigrescens
14. Phallus Impudicus
15. Polyporus Pinicola
16. Psilocybe Caerulescens
17. Russula foetens
18. Secale Cornutum
19. Solanum tuberosum aegrotans
20. Torula Cerevisiae
21. Ustilago Maydis

● Also added should be -

- Thalaspi Bursa - Pastoris (The Shepherd's Purse)-plant belonging to Family Cruciferae. Thalaspi is always invaded by a fungus and its drug picture is due to the fungus parasite and not due to the host plant.

● The lichens, a symbiosis of an alga and fungus in the materia medica are -

1. Cetraria Islandica (Iceland Moss)
2. Chladonia Rangiferina (Reindeer Moss)
3. Sticta Pulmonaria
4. Usnea Barbata.

5

FUNGI

The realm of the fungi is a strange and paradoxical one within the plant kingdom. Fungi have no chlorophyll and therefore live as saprophytes or parasites.

They have no leaves - due to which their metabolism is catabolic. They are composed of mycelial networks, which are made of fine hyphae - thread like columns of simple cells.

From the mycelial networks, arise the fruiting bodies of which the toadstools and mushrooms are very familiar.

The fungi play a major role in decomposing organic matter to inorganic. They can also cause diseases in plants, animals, humans.

SPHERE OF ACTION :

Central Nervous System.[5]

Peripheral Nervous System.[3]

Blood Vessels - Circulation.[3]

Female Sexual Organs - uterus.

Skin.

PATHOGENESIS

1. *CENTRAL NERVOUS SYSTEM.*

   Involves the whole cerebrospinal axis.

   Produces irritation, inflammation and degeneration.

2. *PERIPHERAL NERVOUS SYSTEM.*

   Produces severe multiple neuritis.

3. *BLOOD VESSELS -*

   a) Spasm - ischaemia - gangrene

   b) Dilation - relaxation - haemorrhage.

4. *CONNECTIVE TISSUES* -
Hypertrophy - Fibroids - Tumours Atrophy.
5. *SKIN* -
Inflammation
Exudation
Eczema.

MIASMATIC CLEAVAGE

PSORIC :

Idiopathic epilepsies	(Agaricus)
Idiopathic trembling	(Agaricus)
Trembling after fright	(Agaricus)
Epilepsy after fright	(Agaricus)
Weakness after coitus	(Agaricus)
Fear of cancer.	(Agaricus)
Hay fever - itching of nasopharynx and ears	(Agaricus)

SYCOSIS :

Lymphoid tumour	(Agaricus)
Fibroid Tumour	(Ustilago)
Late in walking, talking	(Agaricus)
Indolence	(Agaricus)
Sciatica < sitting	(Agaricus)
> lying	(Agaricus)
General puffiness	(Bovista)
Pitting Oedema	(Bovista)
Enlarged prostate	(Secale Cor)

TUBERCULAR :

Haemorrhages	
Myelitis	(Secale cor).
Epistaxis	(Agaricus)
Diabetes mellitus	(Bovista)
Fight wants to	(Bovista)
Epistaxis sneezing when	(Bovista)
Bleeding gums sucking when	(Bovista)
Increased sexual desire	(Agaricus, Ustilago)
Varicose veins, ecchymosis, petechiae	(Secale cor).
Passive bleeding, blood - dark, non coagulable	(Secale cor., ustilago)
Tendency to boils and carbuncles	(Secale).
Throws things at people	(Agaricus)
Phthisis	(Agaricus)
Diabetic retinitis	(Secale).
Growing pains in children	(Agaricus).
Memory active	(Agaricus)
Mischievous	(Agaricus)

SYPHILITIC :

Raynaud's disease	(Secale Cor).
Arteriosclerosis.	(Secale cor.)
Paralysis of intestine	(Secale).
Gangrene of foot, toes, senile gangrene	(Secale).
Senile Cataract	(Secale).
Cataract - hard and soft	(Secale).

8

Post diphtheric paralysis	(Secale).
Gangrene of female organs	(Secale).
Angina pectoris	(Secale).
Paralysis of optic nerve	(Bovista).
Ulcers in bowels	(Bovista).

GENERALS

1. TENDENCY TO INVOLUNTARY MOVEMENTS LIKE TWITCHING, JERKING :

   AGARICUS

   * Irregular, angular, uncertain and exaggerated motions - patient reaches too far, staggers or steps too high, drops things, etc.
   * Trembling, twitching, jerkings or fibrillar spasms, esp. of the eyelids and tongue.
   * Twitching ceases during sleep.
   * Head is in constant motion.
   * Twitching of eyelids, Nystagmus.
   * Twitching of muscles about the ears, facial muscles - Grimaces
   * Arms restless, trembling esp. while writing.
   * Uncertain gait.
   * Fingers fly spasmodically while holding things.

   BOVISTA
   * Awkward motions, drops things.
   * Twitching of facial muscles before asthma.

   SECALE COR
   * Twitchings, spasms with fingers apart.
   * Cramps with stiffness and gnawing in single parts.

9

* Tetanic spasms with full consciousness.
* Convulsive jerks and starts in the paralysed limbs.
* Twisting of head to and fro.
* Twitching of abdominal muscles.
* Tingling in back extending to fingers and toes.
* Trembling, staggering or shuffling gait as if feet were dragged along. Toes drawn up.

USTILAGO

* Clonic and tetanic movements.

2. TENDENCY TO DEVELOP PARAESTHESIAS LIKE TINGLING NUMBNESS WITH OR WITH OUT PAIN OR TWITCHING

AGARICUS

* Sensation as if pierced by cold or hot needles.
* Sensation of a cold drop or cold weight on parts.
* Painful twitching followed by coldness and stiffness of parts.
* Neuralgia as if cold needles run through the nerves.
* Shooting and burning along the spine.
* Burning, itching, redness and swelling as if frozen.

BOVISTA

* Multiple neuritis with tingling and numbness.

SECALE COR

* Numbness, insufferable tingling, crawling start-

ing in the face, on the back, in the limbs, in the finger tips > rubbing; on the tip of the tongue and throat.

* Sensation of burning, as if sparks in the whole body.

* Feels as if walking on velvet.

* Formication of the skin.

USTILAGO

* Sensation of boiling water flowing along the back.

3. TENDENCY TO HAEMORRHAGES

BOVISTA

* Nose bleed. Persistent epistaxis in drunkards.

* Bleeding dark, offensive and stringy.

* Metrorrhagia - especially during climaxis.

SECALE COR

* Nose bleed - persistent dark with prostration in old people and drunkards.

* Haemorrhages - thin, foetid, watery, black oozing continuously esp. menses.

* Bleeding of gums.

* Haemorrhage after extraction of teeth.

* Haematemesis.

* Bloody urine.

USTILAGO

* Congestive, passive or slow bleeding, dark watery or in clots forming large black strings.

* Vicarious menstruation.

4. TENDENCY TO INCREASED SEXUAL DESIRE WITH MASTURBATION

   AGARICUS
   * Increased sexual desire in males
   * Sexual excitement in females.

   BOVISTA
   * Increased sexual desire in males.
   * Voluptuous sensation, tingling, coitus - like.
   * Coition aggravates.
   * Dreams - amorous (coition)
   * Dreams - amorous - pollutions with.

   USTILAGO
   * Irresistible desire to masturbate.
   * Erotic fancies.
   * Emissions every night.
   * Emissions even while talking to women.

5. EASY PROSTRATION ESPECIALLY AFTER COITUS OR SEXUAL ABUSE

   AGARICUS
   * Male - Great debility after coition
           - Complaints after sexual debauches.
   * Female - Complaints following coitus
             - Young, hysterical, married women, who faint after coition.

   BOVISTA
   * Reeling and confusion in head after coition.

   USTILAGO
   * Prostration after sexual abuse.

6. TENDENCY TO CATCH COLD, FEELS VERY CHILLY YET AVERSION TO COVERING
   AGARICUS
   * Frequent sneezing without coryza
   * Flow of clear water without coryza.
   * Sneezing after coughing.

   BOVISTA
   * Chilly patient
   * Sensitive to cold.
   * Chilly during pains.

7. ESPECIALLY SUITABLE FOR FEMALES DURING CLIMAXIS
   AGARICUS
   * Bearing down pains esp. after menopause.

   USTILAGO
   * Menorrhagia at climaxis
   * Congestion of various parts esp. during climaxis.
   * Irritability at climaxis.

8. TENDENCY TO FORM NEW GROWTHS
   BOVISTA
   * Para - ovarian cyst.
   * Boil in the right ear with pain and discharge of foetid pus.

   SECALE COR
   * Lymphoid tumors.
   * Boils which mature slowly with green pus.
   * Bloody blisters.

USTILAGO

*   Fibroid tumors.

It has been seen that the group of fungus remedies are useful in cases of mental retardation, as is clearly indicated from the following rubrics.

ABSENT MINDED

AWKWARDNESS

CONFUSED BEHAVIOUR

CONCENTRATION, DIFFICULT

DULLNESS, difficulty in thinking

FORGETFUL

IMBECILITY

INDIFFERENCE, apathy to everything.

INDOLENCE, aversion to work

MEMORY WEAKNESS, done for what has just

MISTAKES, speaking and writing

PROSTRATION of mind, brain fag

SENSES, dull blunted.

● ● ●

4 | HISTORY OF INTRODUCTION OF AGARICUS TO HOMOEOPATHY

Agaricus is a well known poisonous fungus that has been used in Europe, as a FLY POISON for hundreds of years. Cattle are poisoned as well as men by eating it, and it is supposed that flesh is thus rendered unwholesome. The fungus is commonly known for its narcotic value. The usual mode of taking the fungus is to swallow it without chewing. Many times it was used to prepare someone for a deed who would otherwise not do it in a normal state of mind. For instance, the Russians used it for premeditated assassination.

AGARICUS PHALLOIDES : (Amanita Phalloides; Death cup)

Sphere of action: The poison, a toxalbumin resembles the poison of a rattle snake. it acts on red blood corpuscles dissolving them, thereby draining the whole system. The action of the poison is slow, taking atleast 12-20 hours to act.

Characteristic Symptoms: Symptoms in the poisoning cases give a picture of Asiatic Cholera.

Vomiting and purging.

Continuous urging to stool but no gastric, abdominal or rectal pain.

Violent pains in epigastrium < pressure

Intense thirst for cold water.

Dry skin.

Sharp changes from rapid to slow and from slow to rapid breathing, extreme collapse. No cold extrem ities or cramps.

Suppressed urine.

AGARICUS EMETICUS:

Characteristic Symptoms : Severe vertigo, unable to sit or stand.

All symptoms > cold water

Longing for ice water

Sensation as if the stomach hung on threads which would be torn in two.

(Ice cold sweat on face.)

Faintness < moving head, < smelling vinegar.

Violent vomiting

Relation: Acon, Sulphur - Anxiety partially > cold drinks Antim-C, Ars, Bell, Brom, Ferr, Sep, Sulph < Vinegar.

AGARICINUM : (constituent of Polyporus officinale)

Characteristic Symptoms : Useful in following conditions Phthisical & enervating night sweats, profuse perspiration.

(Chorea.)

Pulmonary Emphysema

Dilatation of heart

Erythema.

● ● ●

5 | AGARICUS MUSCARIUS

The word AGARICUS consists of a large genus of fungi consisting of over a thousand species. Hering, therefore considered the word AGARICUS as very vague and thus has given the remedy under AMANITA MUSCARIUS" means "Musca" which means a FLY.

It is also called *FLY AGARIC* because it can kill flies if it is steeped in milk.

It is also known as *SCARLET CAP* because of its red or orange coloured top.

Its *synonyms* are Amanita muscaria, Agaricus imperialis, Amanita citrinus, Agaricus puella, Agaricus Plumboeus, Agaricus Maculatus Pustulatus, Agaricus Verrucosus, Agaricus fulsus depending on its colour which in turn depends on the locality in which it is found. It is called a *TOADSTOOL* - because toads and frogs sit on it and use it as a stool.

In fairy tales it is said that the fairies, gnomes, pixies and all such creatures used these mushrooms to sit on as they had a stalk and a top on which they could sit. They used it as a stool. Thus this mushroom is called a TOADSTOOL.

In Hering's guiding symptoms Agaricus has been given under *AMANITA*. In the Webster's Dictionary, AMANITA is given as any of various usually highly toxic mushrooms of the genus Amanita. The word is derived from the Greek word Amanitai - a fungus.

GEOGRAPHICAL DISTRIBUTION :

It is found in dry places and sandy deserts of Asia and in dry pine woods of Scotland and other parts of N. Europe. Found in Europe, Asia, America, Common in Norway, Sweden, Russia & Lapland.

PROVER : It was first proved by Schreter & E. Staph and published by Staph in 1828 - later Hahnemann and his students proved it and published it in the "Archives" in 1830.

In 1831 Apelt proved the remedy. It was the best proving of all.

PREPARATION : It is prepared from the cap (pileus) of the mushroom. The dried cap is triturated.

It can also be prepared from the stalk (stipes) or the cap - fresh or dried.

If fresh - the stipes and pileus are washed well and the external parts mashed and to it is added equal parts of spirits of wine. It is then kept aside for 3 days and the supernatant fluid is decanted and then attenuated to the 30th dilution.

If the fungus is taken in the dried form - one grain is triturated with 100 grains of sugar of milk.

● ● ●

6 | EVOLUTION OF AGARICUS MIND

KEYWORDS : 1. Alcoholism-Acute and Chronic.

ETIOLOGY :

* It is especially suited for those individuals who have applied their mind in their field of work for a prolonged period without any rest. This is more true of persons engaged as SCIENTISTS or ENGINEERS or it is adapted for those students appearing for professional examinations undergoing long study hours or other professionals like NAVIGATORS or PILOTS. It is also suited to those individuals who have indulged themselves in strong sexual passions for a prolonged period of their life. It could be suited to the sexual partners in their life.

* It is also valuable for those individuals suffering from Manic-depressive psychosis who have become habituated to alcohol.

* Mental over exertion or emotional excitement arising out of the above conditions could be a contributing factor.

Psychoanalysis of the Mental Symptoms:

A common psycho analytical aphorism is "SUPER EGO" is soluble in alcohol"

Alcoholism is extremely effective in anxiety and hence the personalities described above usually turn to alcohol to reduce unconscious stress. Also these individuals have an enhanced need for "power", but feel inadequate to achieve their goals. Alcohol may give such individuals a sense of "release" and power with a sense of achievement.

Rubrics which may indicate this state are :
01. Audacity
02. Courage
03. Delirium - exaltation of strength
04. Delusion - is a great person.
05. Delusion - officer
06. Delusion - things grow small
07. Eccentricity - fancies in
08. Ecstasy
09. Exhilaration, exaltation - in bed
10. Exhilaration, exaltation - at night.
11. Plans - bold.

As alcohol is consumed more during the evening hours many of the symptoms which depict an exaltation of spirits are found to occur in evening or night time.

Rubrics
01. Cheerful, gay - evening.
02. Dullness, difficulty of thinking - evening amel.
03. Dullness, difficulty of thinking - night amel.
04. Excitement, excitable - evening
05. Fancies exaltation of, night.
06. Ideas, abundant - evening
07. Ideas, abundant - bed in
08. Memory, active - evening
09. Thoughts, rush of - evening
10. Thoughts, rush of - night.

At a later stage when a person comes out of the effect of alcohol, an exactly opposite state comes which is characterised by symptoms which are quite opposite to the previous state mentioned above. The symptoms are due to the wearing off of the effect of alcohol which is more in the morning following the consumption of alcohol.

01. Confusion of mind - morning, on waking.
02. Irritability - morning, waking on
03. Morose, cross, ill - humor-morning, waking on
04. Stupefaction, morning.
05. Business, aversion to
06. Chaotic, confused behaviour
07. Forgetful, words while speaking
08. Indifference - business affairs to
09. Indifference - everything.
10. Indifference - work aversion to
11. Senses blunted
12. Thinking, aversion to
13. Work, aversion to, mental
14. Work - impossible.
15. Concentration, difficult studying, reading while.
16. Confusion of mind, reading while.
17. Dullness from mental exertion.
18. Memory weakness of
19. Mistakes in speaking, after exertion.

On further study of provings, it is clearly observed that there is a strong indication of symptoms that suggest alcoholic intoxication characterised by maladaptive behaviour, e.g. loquacity, gregarious, belligerent, etc.

Rubrics :
1. Battles, war, talks of
2. Audacity
3. Loquacity - answers no questions
4. Loquacity - changing quickly from one subject to another.
5. Laughing - involuntary.
6. Laughing - loud.

21

In severe cases of intoxication where the patient becomes extremely disoriented, they experience ávarious delusions and hallucination (visual). There is also an increased psychomotor activity. The patient ámay ádisplay aggressive and impulsive behaviour and may be dangerous for others.

Rubrics :

01. Anger, irascible
02. Delirium - fierce
03. Delirium - raging, raving.
04. Delirium - violent
05. Delusions - vindictive
06. Destructiveness
07. Gestures, violent.
08. Injure himself, frenzy causing him to
09. Kill, desire to
10. Mania, rage with
11. Plans, revengeful.
12. Rage, constant
13. Rage, alternating with religious excitement.
14. Rage, strength increased.
15. Rage, violent
16. Runs, about in most dangerous places.
17. Tears things
18. Threatening.
19. Violence, rage leading to deeds of.

DELUSIONS OF AGARICUS :

1. * Delusion, as if he is ohligod to confess his sins at the gate of hell.

Explanation: The word hell is a noun whose meaning is home of the wicked after death.

In the above situation the person is trying to confess his sins at the gate of hell. This is a delusion whose meaning could be that in reality he may or may not have committed any sin as seen in certain cases of alcoholic intoxication which can produce antegrade amnesia. These periods of amnesia can be particularly distressing because people may fear that they have unknowingly harmed someone or behaved imprudently while intoxicated - "SYNOPSIS OF PSYCHIATRY" by Harold I. Kaplan, M.D. and Benjamin J. Sadock, M.D.

This is a clear cut indication of tremendous GUILT, which could be due to causes described in the beginning.

2. * Delusion, he is commanded to fall on his knees and confess his sins and rip up his bowels by a mushroom.

Here rip up his bowel means to speak without restrain every feeling without any hesitation. One should not get confused here with the other meaning of rip which means split or tear.

The above delusion also indicates the guilt whose explanation is mentioned above.

* There are two other delusions which very characteristically irepresent the Agaricus mind.

They are -
1. Delusion - small hole, appears like a frightful chasm.
2. Delusion - a spoonful of water appears like a lake.

The Agaricus patients tends to magnify all his problems to a great extent. An Agaricus patient comes to the clinic with a very minor problem. But his presentation of the complaint is very exaggerated. His anxiety is out of proportion to the magnitude of the problem.

e.g. 1. He may come with a simple cough and coryza and he may feel that he could be having Tuberculosis.

2. He may come with a glandular enlargement and he would give a big explanation ultimately coming to conclusion that it may be cancer.

3. If the Agaricus patient has a small problem with his boss at office, he may again magnify the whole problem and have all sorts of thoughts like he may be kicked out of his job, or that he may receive a lot of rebuke from his boss.

COMMON DREAMS OF AGARICUS

While studying the dreams of Agaricus one finds that three peculiar dreams convey the feeling. They are as follows :

1. Body, mouth opening impossible

2. Pain in maxillary joint.

3. Unsuccessful efforts, open the mouth to

This could be interpreted as - when one wants to talk, opening of mouth is a must, also when one talks there is some movement at maxillary joint. Here the patient dreams that he is unable to open his mouth because of the pain. This could be interpreted as the person in reality wants to speak up for himself but either he lacks courage or he is repressed due to circumstances. Hence, at the subconscious level this feeling is conveyed in the form of dream.

● ● ●

7

AGARICUS CHILD

The mind of an Agaricus child seems to develop slowly. They are slow in walking, talking and learning. They make mistakes in talking and writing. They have a bad memory. Their speech may be incoherent and jerky. They cannot decide anything for themselves. They will always ask someone to take their decisions. They can also have intense rage with increased strength. This rage can also lead to acts of violence.

Rubrics indicating the above phenomena are :

* Dullness, sluggishness, difficulty of thinking and comprehending - in children.

* Talk - slow learning to

* Walk - late learning to

* Mistakes in speaking

* Mistakes in words - wrong words

* Mistakes in writing

* Memory - weakness of

    " - " - for expressing oneself

    " - " - for - done for what he has just

    " - " - thought for what he has just.

* Irresolution

* Speech - incoherent

    " - by jerks

The Agaricus child will not always present with the above mentioned picture. Another variation would be a child who is very intelligent and bright. Their mind would be very active especially in the evening. They are very curious, always eager to acquire information or knowledge. They will ask many questions to the mother when they come to the clinic. They will not answer any question or refuse to answer. They can be bold - sometimes even shamelessly bold.

They can be very talkative, but never answering questions put to them, always changing quickly from one subject to another.

They like to boast, they can be conceited, always talking about their brilliant and heroic deeds.

They can be quite manipulative, they can mislead you into believing something else. They can also lie sometimes. They grimace while talking especially when they don't want to answer.

They can be self-centered, always thinking about themselves, without any regard for others.

The child could also have an increased sexual desire from an early age.

From the above symptoms we can figure out that the child is mentally perverted. His mind has deviated from what is right. They can obstinately persist in what is wrong. They can be obstinate and self willed also.

The Agaricus child can present with a variety of physical disorders like -

1. Chorea
2. Neuralgia of various types.
3. Epilepsy and epileptiform convulsions.
   Epilepsy from suppressed skin eruptions.
4. Acne Rosacea
5. Spinal irritation.
6. Twitching, jerkings.

8 | CHARACTERISTIC PARTICULARS IN AGARICUS

HEAD
* Coldness of forehead, though it is hot to touch.
* Pain on the right side of head as from a nail,
  < sitting quietly
  > walking about

EYES
* Convulsive, involuntary, pendulum - like movements of the eyes from side to side.
* Twitching, quivering of eyelids < before thunder storm > during sleep.
* Delusion of colours and figures in front of eyes.

EARS
* Chillblains
* Redness of the cartilage
* Extreme itching which feels like burning
* < during menses.

NOSE
* Red tip of nose
* Pain in root of nose during headache
* Prolonged cough ending in sneezing.
* Epistaxis in old people.

FACE
* A stupid, puzzled expression on face.
* Involuntary grimaces
* Repeated blinking of eyes
* (R) sided trigeminal neuralgia.

MOUTH

* Offensive breath, like horse radish
* Teeth- sensitive to touch and feel long.
* Quivering of tongue causing difficulty in speech.

STOMACH

* Empty eructations alternating with hiccoughs
* Eructations tasting like apples or rotten eggs.
* Desires: Salt and salty things.
* Aversion : Bread
            Meat
            Wine
< Cold food
< Cold drinks
> Coffee

ABDOMEN

* Distention of abdomen, flatulence and gurgling
* < before and after breakfast.
* Affection of liver and spleen. Organ pains in joggers.
* Pain in the umbilicus in the morning on waking
* Rumbling after stool < pressure.

RECTUM

* Strong tenesmus before, during and after stool
* Diarrhoea < rising lin the morning. < after eating.
* Diarrhoea with much flatus.
* Constipation - a lot of straining without result.
* Rectum feels unable to expel contents.

URINARY SYSTEM

* Urine feels cold on passing.
* Urgency +
* Milky urine in the afternoon
* Dysuria with a painful coldness and twitching along the left leg.

GENITALIA
* In females, voluptuous itching of the clitoris leading to masturbation.
* Leucorrhoea is copious, dark, bloody and acrid.
* The male genitalia are cold, the testes retracted and painful.

Respiratory System - cough
* Convulsive cough in bronchitis or pneumonia.
* Paroxysmal coughing ending in sneezing.
* Ball like expectoration.

CHEST
* Palpitations are worse in the evening and after stool.

BACK
* Back is very sensitive especially between the scapulae.
* Sensation of cold water being poured over the parts.
* Lumbago, Sciatica.
< Motion
< trying to raise the thigh while sitting.
< raising himself from the bed.
> lying down.
* Sensation of tension in the back.
< Standing
< stretching
< touch.

EXTREMITIES
* Difficulty in coordinating the movements
* Clumsy and awkward when handling things.
* Paralytic weakness of the lower limbs during pregnancy.
* Twitching in the nates.
* Coldness in spots - cold spot felt in the elbow.

SKIN
* Angioneurotic oedema.
* Easy ecchymosis.
* Burning, itching and redness
* Coldness in spots
* Sensation as if frost bitten.

SLEEP
* Starting on falling asleep.
* Ineffectual, frequent yawning followed by nervous laughter.

● ● ●

9

ALCOHOLISM OF
AGARICUS

* Garrulousness   : Dementia
(habitually, often excess : Loquacity - answers no
ively talkative)   questions but - chang-
                            ing quickly from one-
                            subject to another.
                      : Answers-sings, talks, but
                            will not answer ques-
                            tions.
* Aggressiveness   : Anger, irascibility
                      : Injure   himself-frenzy
                            causing him to injure
                            himself.
                      : Kill, desire to
                      : Mutilating his body.
                      : Rage, fury-alternating
                            with religious excitement
                               - constant
                               - during drunkenness
                               - strength increased
                               - violent.
                      : Violent, vehement
                               - deeds of violence,
                                 rage, leading to
* Excessive activity   : Restlessness
                               - evening
                               - midnight, after 3h.
                               - internal
                               - night, in a dream.

	:	Runs about - dangerous places, in most

MOTOR PERFORMANCE

* Standing posture,	:	Stiff all over
* Control of speech and eye	:	Uncertain gait
movement,	:	Stumbles over everything in the way
* Highly organized and complex motor skills	:	Trembling of the hands
- are adversely affected	:	Paralysis of lower limb
	:	Tearing painful contraction in the calves
	:	Paralysis of upper limb and lower limb - from incipient softening of spinal cord.

MENTAL FUNCTION

* Hearing, concentration attention affected.	:	Concentration difficult - studying reading, etc. while.
	:	Concentration difficult - learns with difficulty.
	:	Development of children arrested
	:	Dullness, sluggishness, difficulty of thinking and comprehending.

ALCOHOLIC INTOXICATION

* Outburst of blind fury	:	Anger, irascibility
with assaultive and	:	Battles, war talks of

destructive behaviour	:	Insanity, strength increased with
	:	Kill desire to
	:	Mania, rage with
	:	Rage - constant
		- drunkenness during
		- strength increased
		- violent
	:	Violent, vehement
		- deeds of violence, rage leading to
	:	Tears things.
* Gross social indiscretions	:	Audacity (shamelessly bold)
	:	Malicious.

● ● ●

10 DERMATOLOGY OF AGARICUS

A. Angioneurotic Oedema :

1. *Causation* : Alcoholism, Grief, Fright, Sexual excess.

2. *Appearance* : The affected part appears bright red.

3. *Sensations* : Severe burning and itching; itching changes the place on scratch ing.

B. Frost bites -

1. *Causation* : Exposure to severe cold weather.

2. *Appearance* : Bluish red discolouration.

3. *Sensations* : Burning and itching - Sensation as if cold needles are pricking.

C. Easy Ecchymosis -

D. Profuse oily perspiration; -

E. Modalities -

* Most of the symptoms are worse especially after coitus.

* The chilliness is worse in open air, drafts, lifting the clothes.

OPHTHALMOLOGY OF AGARICUS

Affections of eyelids -

*   Twitching of eyelids - < before a thunder-storm.

*   Margins of the lid-red, it itches, burns and agglutinates

*   Inner angles very red

*   Gum in canthi, viscid yellow.

*   Narrowing of space between eyelids.

Affections of vision -

*   Double vision.

*   Vision dim as from a mist, after looking long at any object while reading.

*   Flickering before the eyes while writing.

*   Muscae volitantes.

*   Asthenopia from prolonged strain.

*   Short sighted.

Affections of muscles & nerves -

*   Nystagmus.

● ● ●

12 SEXUALITY OF AGARICUS

* Sexually Agaricus is easily excitable, intense and overactive. The desire is excessive in the morning.

* After coition
  - GREAT DEBILITY
  - PROFUSE SWEAT
  - BURNING AND ITCHING OF THE SKIN.
  - TENSION and PRESSURE UNDER RIBS.
  - DEPRESSED.

* The mental symptoms of extreme anxiety and fear are ameliorated temporarily after sexual intercourse.

* Seminal emissions without dreams

* After an emission great debility and lassitude.

* Pains and weakness in the thighs after emission.

* Excessive masturbation from reading pornographic materials or viewing blue films.

* They search for easy pleasure without much responsibility.

● ● ●

13 CHOREA OF AGARICUS

MIND

*	Nagging other members of the family	: Obstinate
*	Suspicious	: - -
*	Irritable	: Irritable, waking on.
		Irritable, coition after
*	Eccentric	: Dancing, grotesque
		: Gestures, strange attitudes and position of head.
		: Eccentricity in fancies.
*	Religious, excessive	: - -
*	False sense of superiority	: Egotism, reciting their exploits
		: Delusion - officer he is an.
		- great person, he is.
		- Plans - bold.
*	Poor self control	: Confusion of mind
		- intoxicated as if
		- reading, while
		- waking, on
		- walking, on
		: Chaotic
		: Concentration, difficult

- studying while
- learns with difficulty.

: Injure himself, frenzy causing him to injure himself.

: Mutilating his body

: Insanity with increased strength.

: Indifference apathy-aversion to work.
- business affairs to everything to

* Promiscuity   : Amorous

Lascivious

. Lustful

* Fits of despondency   : Sadness, despondency, dejection
- coition after
- headache, during
- masturbation, from
- pollutions, from
- sexual excesses from
- trifles, about.

* Mood, disorder of   : Mood, changeable, variable

; Morose, cross - on waking

: Sulky

● ● ●

14 MULTIPLE SCLEROSIS IN AGARICUS

MULTIPLE SCLEROSIS   **AGARICUS**

Precipitating Factors :
* Infection
* Trauma (physical injury)
* Pregnancy

Clinical Symptoms and Signs

1) *Weakness, numbness :   * Weakness (1703)
                              * Numbness -affected
                                parts (1637)
                              * Numbness-extremi
                                ties (1208)
                                - forearms, hands
                                  (1213)
                                - hips, legs (1214)
                              * Tingling-hands.
                                - lower limbs.

2) Tight band sensation
   around trunk and
   extremities   : Sensation of constric-
                           tion - elbow, shoulder
                           (1144)

3) * Dragging or poor control of one or both legs : *Awkwardness-lower limbs (1132)

-stumbles when walking (1132)

* In co-ordination : * Ataxia (1132)

04) Retrobulbar optic neuritis : Inflammation-optic nerve (368)

05) Partial or total loss of vision : Loss of vision (409)

06) Hemianopia : Hemianopia (408)
07) Scotoma - macular area : Scotoma (44)
08) Brain stem S/s-Diplopia: Diplopia (405)
09) Vertigo, vomiting : Vertigo (213)
10) Cerebellar symptoms like scanning speech, Nystagmus : Eye - pendulum like motion (372)

11) * Intentional tremors-drunkards : * Trembling - upper limbs (1369)

* Incoordination : - hands (1370)

- lower limbs (1371)
12) Bladder symptoms - : Bladder- frequent urge (807)

* Hesitancy, urgency, frequency, incontinence, retention : - retention (804)
13) Abrupt attacks of

Neurologic deficits
- dysarthria and ataxia
- paroxysmal pain and dysesthesia
- flashing lights and tonic flexion of wrist and elbow.

: * Speech-difficult (556)

14) Unusually severe and transient fatigue is another peculiar symptom of multiple sclerosis

: Weakness - tremulous (1713)

15) Mental Symptoms in multiple sclerosis are euphoria, a pathological symptom

: * Ecstasy (91)
: * Cheerful (26)
: * Sadness (168)

- Cheerfulness or elation (stupid indifference, morbid, optimism)

: Sadness-morning(169)
- evening (169)

16) Recurrent seizures as a result of lesions of cerebral cortex

: Convulsions (1568)

● ● ●

41

15 CHILBLAINS

AGARICUS		PETROLEUM
Common Symptoms		
Burning		
Itching		
Redness		
Swelling		
< Winter		
> Summer		
* Skin - dry (+)	:	* Skin - dry (++++)
* Skin - rough (+)	:	* Skin - rough (++++)
* -	:	* Skin - Sensitive < touch of clothes
* -	:	* Easy bleeding
* Skin - cracks-more superficial :	:	* Skin- cracks-much more deep.
-	:	* Itching is so violent that one must scratch until it bleeds.
	·	* Parts become cold after itching
* Itching changes place on scratching	:	-
		* If Chilblains are suppressed they cause diarrhoea.

● ● ●

16 COMPLAINTS APPEAR DIAGONALLY

AGARICUS

Symptoms appear at the same time on the opposite sides of the body but diagonally (Right upper and left lower or vice versa). Pain in right arm and left leg.

Here also the neurological pathology is prominent.

On one side there is tingling numbness or cold needle sensation and on the other side one gets chorea, twitching and convulsions.

STRAMONIUM

Complains appear diagonally, upper left and lower right. These diagonal affections are usually neurological in nature where one side is paralysed and the other has convulsions. One side is paralysed and the other has trembling or there can be rheumatic affections that is involvement of hip joint on one side and shoulder joint on opposite side.

● ● ●

17 FEAR OF CANCER

AGARICUS

Extreme anxiety about health. Preoccupied with the diseases of those around them.

As a result of fear of cancer they will go through sleepless nights.

The above fear is triggered by any trivial pain anywhere in the body and then the patient may exaggerate and insist on a detailed physical and laboratory investigation.

KALI ARS

This remedy has fear of cancer but it is not focused only on one disease. It is focused also on other diseases, ischaemic heart disease, stroke, etc.

These fears are known to culminate in real panic attacks which are characterised by anxiety with restlessness, tossing about in bed or the patient may get up from sleep startled, with difficulty in breathing, trembling of the limbs, feels very chilly.

The above attack usually comes between 1.00 and 3.00 A.M.

● ● ●

18 PERIPHERAL NEURITIS

AGARICUS	ARS-ALB
Sensation :	
Icy cold needles or sen :	Hot needles.
sation of cold weight on	Tingling in fingers.
the parts	
Itching of the affected part :	Fingers cannot be extended.
as if frozen.	
< COLD AIR :	Restless feet
< freezing air :	Paraesthesia > hot application
< coitus	> hot wraps
< morning :	< midnight
< alcohol :	< after midnight
A/F *coition :	< cold damp weather
*Sexual excesses :	< tobacco
*alcoholism :	A/F Ptomaine poisoning, grief, fright, burns, quinine poisoning.

● ● ●

19

CHOREA

AGARICUS

Chorea from simple motion
and jerks of single muscles
to dancing of whole body.
Headaches of those subject
to chorea.

Grimaces; distortion of the
mouth
> during sleep

< before thunderstorm

< coition

ZINCUM

: Chorea especially of
the extremities

: < during sleep

: < during dentition

: < stimulants.

CHOREA

AGARICUS

* Chorea especially of
eye-lids and tongue

A/F

- Depletion of energy as
a consequence of sexual
excesses

MYGALE LASIODORA

: * Chorea especially of
upper parts i.e.
muscles of the face,
eyes and eyelids.

A/F

: -

- Fear originating from
  death of loved ones,
  grief, vexation : -

DIRECTION:

- Chorea especially on right
  arm and left leg or left
  side of the face

TYPE:

- A few muscle fibres quiver
  quite frequently and change
  place quickly, driving the
  patient crazy

MODALITIES

< before thunderstorm

< alcohol

< coition

> during sleep

DIRECTION

: - Chorea especially on
  the right side.

TYPE:

: - Mouth and eyes open
  in rapid succession,
  words are jerked out
  in the effort to talk.

MODALITIES

: < morning > during
  sleep.

● ● ●

20

SPINAL SYMPTOMS

AGARICUS

A/F

- Depletion of energy as a consequence of sexual excesses

- Fear - originating from death of loved ones
- Grief
- Vexation

CONVULSIONS

< After coitus

< Suppressed milk

< After being scolded or punished

Convulsions from suppressed eruptions.

CONCOMITANT

- Physical strength increased

ZINCUM MET

A/F

: - Fright
- Suppressed eruptions

: - Suppressed discharges

: - Spinal injury

CONVULSIONS

: - During dentition

: - Convulsions from fright

: - Automatic motion of one hand and head

: - With pale face

: - No heat-no increase in temperature

: - Rolling of the eyes

: - Grinding of the teeth

TREMBLING

- Involuntary movements while awake, cease during sleep
- Arms restless

TREMBLING

: - Fidgety feet
: - Trembling of hands when writing during menses

TWITCHING, JERKING

- Painful twitching, then the parts become stiff and cold

TWITCHING, JERKING

: < night
: < during sleep

PARAESTHESIA

(S) as if pierced by needles of ice or hot needles

- Pains are accompanied by (S) of coldness, numbness & tingling

- Sensitiveness of the spine to touch - < open air, < sitting, < pressure, < touch

PARAESTHESIA

: - Cannot bear back touched

: - Burning along spine < sitting

: - Transverse pains in the limbs never length - wise

- Formication of feet and back which prevents sleep > rubbing > pressure

- Numbness of the legs on crossing them

: - One part numb, another sensitive.

49

PARALYSIS

- Uncertain gait, stumbles
  over everything in the way :

PARALYSIS

- Descending paralysis

- Stumbling, spastic gait

- Totters while walking especially in the dark with closed eyes.

MODALITIES

< Walking in open air

< alcohol

< cold air es

< before thunderstorm

< coition

< open air

> warmth in bed

> slow motion

MODALITIES

: < lying down

: < suppressed eruptions

: < suppressed discharg-

: < suppressed menses

: > free discharges

: > menses

: > motion

: > hard pressure

> rubbing

> appearance of erup-tions

21 AWKWARDNESS DROPS THINGS

AGARICUS
* Trembling and twitchings in different parts of the extremities which makes one prone to awkward postures, movement and finally difficulty in balancing.
* Difficulty in coordinating the movements of the extremities. He may overstretch his legs, reaching too far, too high with irregular angular motion when ascending or descending stairs. He is clumsy and awkward when handling things, stumbles when walking.

    His fingers may fly open spasmodically for no apparent reason, causing him to drop whatever he is holding.

BOVISTA
* Awkwardness is basically due to sexual excesses.
* Awkward in speech: stuttering and stammering while reading.

    - action: drops things.

APIS
* Paralyses of the right side after excessive grief.
* There is a definite tendency to paralysis in extremities. The whole nervous system is under a paralytic influence in scarlatina.
* One side paralysed, the other twitching or convulsing. The extremities become heavy, stiff and powerless. Upper extremities perfectly powerless. Cannot take hold of anything. Has to be fed (in spinal disease).

● ● ●

22 DELAYED MILESTONES

AGARICUS
* Slow in walking, talking and learning.
* Mind seems to develop slowly so at a later stage they make mistakes in talking and writing.
* They have a very poor memory, and are slow in comprehending as a result they become extremely dependant on their parents.

BARYTA CARB
* Late in learning to walk, talk, etc.
* Due to idiocy they cannot be taught anything. They are weak mentally as well as physically.
* They usually suffer from single effects. i.e. out of various mile stones, all may not be delayed, few are developed on time while one particular area of development is delayed.
* Also because of the poor confidence that the child has, he fails to learn to walk.

CALCAREA CARB
* Lack of calcium and phosphate metabolism.
* Lack of bone forming substances.
* Pathological fractures of bones.
* Crooked and deformed extremities.
* Easy fracture of bones.

NATRUM MUR
* These children are quite closed. They make a lot of mistakes in speaking, in what they do not intend to utter.
* They have a strong need for affection and hence whenever they do not get the same they are emotionally effected and hence they are late in talking.
* Heavy and difficult speech.

(Ankles are weak and turn easily as described by Dr. Nash). Hence the baby is late in learning to walk.

23 AGGRAVATION AFTER COITUS

AGARICUS

Mostly symptoms related to CNS like chorea, trembling, twitching are aggravated after coitus.

Also psychologically the patient faints after every sexual intercourse. This is due to over-excitement. However anxiety and fear are ameliorated some time after intercourse.

KALI CARB

Coitus aggravates the whole organism from the head to foot producing severe prostration especially of the muscles of the eyes, weakness of the knees, sleeplessness. The prostration is so severe that it remains for 2-3 days after coitus.

AGARICUS   **BUFO**

COMMON

Absentminded, unobserving

A/F Fright

Childish behaviour

Company aversion to

Concentration difficult

Confusion of mind - morning
                  - eating after
                     intoxicated as if

Deceitful, sly.

Delirium tremens, mania-a-potu.

Destructiveness.

Dipsomania, alcoholism.

Fancies, exaltation of

Fear - of impending disease
      - of misfortune.

Foolish behaviour

Hysteria

Idiocy

Imbecility

Irresolution, indecision
Irritability - morning waking on
Lascivious, lustful
Laughing
Malicious, spiteful, vindictive.
Memory weakness for done for what has just.
Mistakes speaking in, words using wrong.
Mood changeable, variable
Morose, cross, fretful, ill-humor, peevish
Offended easily, takes everything in bad part.
Prostration of mind, mental exhaustion, brain fag
Rage, fury,
Runs about
Shrieking - sleep during
Sighing
Starting, startled
Stupefaction as if intoxicated

AGARICUS   **BUFO**

DIFFERENCE

Despair + Rage bordering on	:	Despair
Dipsomania +++	:	+
Dullness, children in	:	-
Egotism, reciting their exploits	:	-
Embraces his companions	:	-
Escape attempts to	:	-

Exhilaration++	:	-
Fear-of cancer	:	Fear-of infection
- of suffocation at night	:	- in a crowd
Gestures - grasping or reaching at something, at flocks, carphologia	:	Gestures-grasping genitals delirium during
Grimaces, jesting	:	Giggling
Indolence - aversion to work	:	Impatience
Kisses hands his companions	:	- -
Mischievous	:	- -
Mutilating his body	:	- -
-	:	Music, < aversion to
-	:	Obscene, lewd talk
Obstinate, headstrong	:	- -
Occupation, diversion >	:	- -
Pities himself	:	- -
Proportion, sense of disturbed	:	- -
Rage, fury + 3	:	Rage, fury + 1
- constant	:	- -
- strength increased	:	- -
Runs about dangerous places in most	:	Runs about
Sensitive - noise, talking, of	:	Sensitive - music to, noise to
--	:	Shamelessness

--	:	Shrieking - uncon-sciousness until
Speech - incoherent	:	Speech - nonsensical
- jerks by	:	- unintelligible
- respectful	:	- foolish
- merry, wandering	:	- -
Strangers - spoken to averse to being	:	Strangers - presence of <
Starting, startled	:	Starting startled
- jerking or twitching	:	- sleep during
- ceasing on falling asleep	:	- easy
--	:	Strikes desire to
Think aversion to, complains of	:	Symptoms, magnifies her.
Throws things at persons	:	Ugly (Behaviour)
Unconsciousness - coition after	:	Unconsciousness-convulsions after.
Verses makes	:	- -
Whistling	:	- -

● ● ●

25 SECALE CORNUTUM MIND

After one studies the original provings of Secale one clearly understands that the remedy is more suitable for a woman who is in childbed or a woman who has undergone an abortion.

The emotional life of such a person is in severe turmoil and the close relatives of the patient are overtly and covertly responsible for the same. This state is represented very clearly in the form of the following rubrics.

* Forsakes relations.
* Contemptuous relations for
* Delirium, abandons relatives.
* Mocking, relatives at his.

The anger that is built up due to this turmoil is expressed in the form of severe degree of violence characterised by the following rubrics.

* Mania, with rage.
* Mania, with deeds of violence.
* Rage, had to be chained.
* Rage, kill people tries to
* Rage, biting with
* Destructiveness.
* Delirium, violent
* Fight, wants to

One can also study an important delusion in Secale.

* Delusion, room is like the foam of a troubled sea.

Here, troubled sea indicates the emotional turmoil

in the domestic life of the patient. It is during this phase that the person tries to express her innermost feelings of resentment against her relatives. Rubrics of this state are given above.

Secale is also adapted to persons who are prone to suffer from Manic Depressive Psychosis. It arises after prolonged use of alcohol, or sexual excesses. During mania the following gestures are important to observe as given in the rubris below.

* Gestures, clapping overhead.

* Gestures, fingers spread apart.

* Gestures, grasping genitals during spasms.

The person can become violent which is characterised by

* Delirium, raging & raving.

* Delirium, maniacal

* Mania, rage with

* Rage, kill people tries to

* Rage, malicious.

* Tears himself.

These attacks of Manic Depressive Psychosis are concentrated around post the partum period and lactation. It is aggravated by the following conditions :

* Puerperal fever

* Suppression of milk.

* Prolonged after pains.

The person during this state also loses her modesty as indicated by

* Naked, wants to be

* Naked, wants to be, delirium in

* Shamelessness

* Exposes the person

59

* Tears her genitals
* Delirium, erotic
* Indifference exposure of her person, to
* Dresses indecently

Attempts of suicide are also present during this state as indicated by

* Suicidal disposition
  " " by drowning
  " " throwing himself from height.
* Jumping river impulse to jump into the

● ● ●

26 BOVISTA LYCOPERDON

- " PUFF BALL "

Bovista, buffen or puffen, puff + fist, to break wind; Lycoperdon, lukos, wolf + perdo, I break wind.

Bovista, the common European puff ball, was first proved by Hartlaub, one of Hahnemann's fellow provers, in 1828. The entire fungus is used to prepare the tincture.

CHARACTERISTIC GENERALS:

* General puffiness, bloated condition of body surface which produces easy indentation with blunt instruments (scissors, etc.)

* Laxity of various tissues.

* Enlarged or swollen feeling in head, heart, etc.

* Effects of application of tar locally.

* Chilly person, sensitive to cold. Feels chilly during pains.

* Tough, stringy, tenacious discharges.

* Most of the physical complaints are worse before and during menses.

● ● ●

27 EVOLUTION OF THE MIND OF BOVISTA LYCOPERDON

Typically Bovista patients are on border line between normal intelligence and mental retardation as with evolution of the mind compared to other fungi, the patient is of subnormal intelligence. This could be due to either defects of development or due to premature degeneration.

The following rubrics clearly indicate the above -

1. Imbecility
2. Senses - blunted, dull.
3. Ideas - deficiency of
4. Concentration - difficult ; attention, cannot fix.
5. Chaotic, confused behaviour.
6. Looking, sky, at, reason, without
7. Confusion of mind.
8. Absent minded
9. Memory - weakness of
10. Mistakes - localities in
             - space and time, in
             - speaking, in
             - writing in
11. Awkwardness.

With this mental retardation they have like other fungi, ailments from sexual excesses and coitus aggravates.

The most unique thing about Bovista patient is that they are not shy to discuss them openly or they are too naive, too frank to understand that basically discussing sex in open is considered taboo in most of the sections of to-days society. They very frankly discuss their sexual problems in front of the doctor in the very first visit.

The following rubrics indicate the frankness.

1. Loquacity - open hearted
2. Audacity
3. Naive
4. Truth tells the plain.

The increased desire for sex is indicated by the following rubrics:

1. Lustful
2. Ailments from sexual excess
3. Dreams - amorous
4. Dreams - Snakes, of (Snake signifies sexual energy and impulse. It can also signify that the person has got frustrated sexual impulses).

Such frankness and open heartedness is often not appreciated in this world, rather this patient is laughed at and criticized as represented in their dreams and mind.

DREAMS - frightful (anxious)
    - arrest - imprisonment (prisoner)
    - vexations.

MENTAL SYMPTOMS - 1. Fear of Pins.
    2. Fear of sharp instruments.

Here fear of pins and sharp pointed instruments indicates fingers pointed at him for being so frank and naive.

3. Fight - wants to
4. Cursing, swearing
5. Quarrelsome.
6. Irritability - takes everything in bad part.

This does not affect the patient and he continues to behave in the same way till a stage comes when he develops complete a cut-off from the society as indicated in the following rubrics:

1. Aversion, to company
2. Aversion, everything to
3. Indifference, apathy - company, society, while in
   - everything to
   - life, to
4. Jesting - aversion to

This state can lead to developing habits like alcohol.

The following rubrics indicate it.
   * Confusion of mind - wine after.
   * Dipsomania

● ● ●

28   CHARACTERISTIC PARTICULARS IN BOVISTA

VERTIGO

Vertigo and momentarily unconscious in morning.
Sudden attacks of vertigo while standing.
< morning.
< standing.

HEAD

Sensation as if head were enlarging especially occiput.
Deep-seated pains in the brain.
Feeling as if head were too large
Digestive headache.
Staggering, confusion and numbness in head
< coition.
< early morning
< open air
< lying
< raising up
Itching of scalp < warmth
                < getting warm
Itching extending to the nape of neck.

EYES

Loss of vision from paralysis of optic nerve.
Eyes look weak and dim.
Staring at one point.
Objects seem nearer than they are.

EARS

Boil in right ear.

Pain < swallowing.

Hearing indistinct.

Discharge - fetid pus.

NOSE

Epistaxis < early morning
  < during sleep

Few drops of blood escape from the nose on sneezing, or blowing the nose. Epistaxis from traumatism.

Epistaxis associated with menstrual irregularity.

Discharge - stringy, tough

Cannot breathe through the nose.

FACE

Scurf & crusts about the nostrils and corners of mouth. Chapped lips.

Acne < summer
  < due to cosmetics.

Pale swelling of upper lip.

Frequent alternations of colour.

MOUTH

Stammering

Bleeding of gums on sucking them.

Violent aching in carious teeth > Open air
  > warmth
  < evening

Increased salivation

Offensive odour from mouth.

Haemorrhage after extraction of teeth.

STOMACH

Nausea > breakfast.

Sensation as of a lump of ice in the stomach
Excessive hunger
Desire for cold drinks afternoons and evenings.
Nausea and chilliness, the whole forenoon.

ABDOMEN

Intolerance of tight clothing around waist.
Colic > eating
     > bending double
Cutting colic < rest, flatulent colic
Colic with red urine
Chilliness especially after stool.
Ulceration in bowels.

RECTUM

Chronic diarrhoea of old people
< night
< early morning.
Diarrhoea < before menses.
         < during menses.
First portion of stool is hard; latter part thin and watery.

URINARY SYSTEM

Diabetes Mellitus
Desire to urinate, immediately after urination.

MALE

Excessive sexual desire.
Vertigo and confusion of head after coition.

FEMALE

Menses too early and profuse
< night
> motion
Menses flowed for most part only at night
Traces of menses between menstruation.

Leucorrhoea acrid, thick, tough, greenish
Stains linen green in spots.
Leucorrhoea a few days before or a few days after the menses. Leucorrhoea like the white of an egg.

RESPIRATORY SYSTEM

Shortness of breath from least exertion.
Cutting pain in tongue before asthma.
Viscid expectoration.

HEART

Visible palpitations of old maids
Palpitation as if heart working water.
Palpitations < bathing
           < excitement
           < during menses
           < eating.
PalpitationS & restlessness, nausea and headache.

BACK

Tip of coccyx itches intolerably.
Must scratch until parts become raw and sore
Pain and stiffness of the back after stooping.

EXTREMITIES

Unusually deep impression on finger from blunt instruments. Great weakness of all joints
Clumsiness with her hands, drops things.
Moist eczema on the back of the hand.
Oedema in joints after fractures.
Sensation in the wrist joint as if sprained.

SLEEP

Great drowsiness < afternoon
              < early morning
              < after eating.

FEVER

Chill

Predominates.

Chill with pain

Chill every day from 7 to 10.00 P.M.

Chilliness all night and shivering in the back.

Chills with thirst.

Heat

Heat with thirst.

Anxiety and restlessness

Sweat in morning.

SKIN

Urticaria on excitement

Itching on getting warm

Eczema, moist formation of thick crusts.

Eczema, red, burns, itches

Tetters, dry appearing in hot weather - during full moon.

Herpes of lower extremities.

MODALITIES

< Before & during menses

< Getting warm.

< Hot weather

< Cold food.

> Bending double

> Hot food.

● ● ●

BOVISTA

* Skin indented easily with pressure

* Herpes-dry, appearing in hot weather and during full moon especially of lower extremities.

* Urticaria on excitement associated with rheumatic lameness, palpitations and diarrhoea. Urticaria on waking in the morning and worse from bathing.

* Eczema associated with thick crusts or scab formation with pus beneath associated with burning and itching.

* Modalities:

< Morning

< Warm weather

< getting warm

< washing.

APIS

* Tensed oedema of the skin, so tense that it seems that the skin will tear. Skin is very sensitive to touch.

* Angio neurotic oedema especially involving the face & lips. Swelling is pink and waxy.

* Urticaria-bright, red, nodular lesions with severe burning. Urticaria aftor violent exercise.

* Eczema with marked swelling .

* Modalities :

< Warmth

< closed room

> cold application

DULCAMARA

* Oedema after ague, rheumatism or scarlet fever.
* Warts-flat and smooth
* Urticaria associated with gastric derangements. Large wheals. Urticaria comes on in the beginning of winter worse-cold air-undressing.
* Eczema < before menses
         < during menses
(especially of face, genitals, hands. Eruptions with thick yellowish brown crusts).
* Modalities:
         < Suppressed eruptions
         < Warmth
         > cold

● ● ●

71

BOVISTA
* Oozing haemorrhages due to relaxation of the capillary system.
* Modalities:
  < night

SECALE COR
* Passive haemorrhage in feeble cachectic females Continuous oozing of thin, foetid watery black blood.
* Bleeding is mainly uterine or in the form of epistaxis or purpura.
* Nose bleed-Dark oozing with great prostration in old people, drunkards or young women.
* Small wounds bleed much
* Concomitant :
  Extensive exhaustion

USTILAGO
* Passive haemorrhage, slow oozing or cloto Dluud is dark but watery or bright red.
* Bleeding is mainly uterine
* Vicarious bleeding from lungs and bowels.
* Modalities:
  < Slightest provocation.

● ● ●

31 MENSTRUAL SYMPTOMS

BOVISTA

* Too early

Metrorrhagia

* Too profuse
< night
> motion
* Profuse flow especially early morning. Scanty during the day and night followed for most part only at night

* Traces of menses between menstruation

* Leucorrhoea
Acrid, thick, tough, green staining green spots on linen

< after menses, < walking

* Concomitant

Soreness of pubes during menses

AMBRA GRISEA

: * Too early

: * Too profuse
: < Lying down
: -   -
: *Discharge of blood between periods, at every little accident, after hard stools, walking a little longer.

: -   -

: * Leucorrhoea Bluish
:   < night.
: * Concomitant
: Itching of Peudendum
    < during urination.

● ● ●

73